Pawsome Palate

Nutritious Homemade Recipes for Vibrant Pets

Freedom - Chapter Publishing

Table of Contents

Disclaimer

Always consult with a veterinarian or pet nutritionist before making any significant changes to your pet's diet.

This book is intended to serve as a general guide, and should always be adapted to the specific needs of individual pets.

Introduction

We have all witnessed how diet has gained major relevance within the past few years. Approaching wellness with fresh foods as our biggest ally is now more popular than ever, and new information about the benefits of natural and balanced nutrition pops up non-stop. It is not hard to imagine that the same principle—nourishing your body with the best foods—works just as well on our pets as it does on us.

For decades, we've been told that there is no better way to feed our pets than with dry food pellets, which are presented by many as the ultimate food, the one and only that can provide our beloved pets with the nutrients they need. The pet food industry is not properly controlled by the FDA, which leads to manufacturers using many ingredients and "fillers" that are not exactly beneficial to our pets in the long run. Pet food is designed to be palatable and contribute to nourishment, but there's definitely a way to step up the feeding game through homemade meals. A home-cooked meal made with fresh ingredients that are actually healthy for our pets will definitely be much more beneficial.

If we compare this to the way human wellness works, we can definitely trace elements like fresh ingredients, simple preparations, and adequate portions and translate that into an awesome diet that allows pets to thrive. There is no denying that homemade diets require far more effort, but nothing that cannot be achieved by understanding the basics of cooking and individualized meal planning, which is what you're here for!

If you ask me, it is quite unfortunate that the influence of homemade meals on our pet's health is not the bigger topic of research, but still, enough studies have been performed so far to know that the results are pretty promising. To name a few benefits, fresh natural meals can prevent several medical conditions—which leads to an increase in longevity—cases of allergies improve, digestion works much better, pets with obesity problems reach their optimal weight in a healthy way, mobility problems decrease, among other benefits for your furry friend.

But your pet is not the only one that'll benefit from this new lifestyle! I can't be the only one who knows the struggle of a picky eater, and if you have been there too, you'll be glad to learn that homemade meals are the best way to help your picky eater try new foods. Hey, I would be tired of eating the same food every day, wouldn't you? Providing them with nourishing and delicious food will also help you continue to bond with your beloved pet, as they will certainly appreciate having meals that they enjoy. Our little ones are smart, and they know we're doing this because we love them! Giving your pet homemade meals turns eating into an inevitably positive experience, and many owners even have some fun while cooking.

Once you decide to take the leap, it is important that you learn how to make meals that accommodate your pet's specific needs, which starts with choosing the right ingredients. To start off, we can state that fresh high-quality ingredients are a must, in order to fulfill your furry friend's nutritional needs, then the right combinations must be carefully prepared, and finally hand out the correct portions.

Throughout this book, we will break down everything there is to know about pet nutrition. From the nutritional needs of popular domestic animals to choosing ingredients, cooking techniques, and delicious recipes for your pets. We'll also debunk common needs regarding homemade diets as you learn the science behind the creation of the best meals. Buckle up, and let's get right to it.

Chapter 1:

Understanding Pet Nutrition

It is no surprise that pet nutrition is an incredibly broad topic to cover, and even more so when we consider the nutritional needs of different species, breeds, and ages. For example, it is clear that you wouldn't feed the same food to a cat as you would to a dog. Just like a puppy and a senior have different requirements, so do animals that are very active versus those with a more sedentary life. However, once you get a hold of it, sustaining a proper diet becomes very simple, as you only need to know your proportions. This means that, depending on your pet's needs, you'll need to provide a specific amount of protein, carbohydrates, and fats. At the same time, micronutrients like vitamins and minerals need to be part of their diet, helping your pet feel happy and energized.

In this chapter, you'll learn how to select the right ingredients, proportions, and nutrients for your pet's needs according to their species, breed, age, and activity level. We will also talk about sources of macro and micronutrients, as well as the importance of portion control. So how exactly do we know what our pets need? Let's begin by understanding the importance of animal physiology.

Specific Nutrition for Specific Pets

Isn't it amazing how our lives are intertwined with so many wonderful animals? This is definitely their world and we just live in it, and there are certain species that we have grown particularly close to. Dogs, cats, rabbits, guinea pigs, and birds are just some of the many pets that have become part of our families, and it is important to know what each of them needs to thrive.

First of all, I think we can agree that all animals require certain nutrients, regardless of their age or species. Things like protein, fiber, antioxidants, minerals, or probiotics are indispensable in a good diet, no matter what kind of pet you own, with the amount of it being the biggest variable. In nature—or at any given space and time where there's no kibble—animals hunt, gather or graze, and they have an instinct that helps them find the right sources of nutrients. When they depend on us, it is now our duty to provide the right food for them, taking their innate needs into consideration.

For example, domestic animals like dogs and cats were practically born to live alongside humans, but they are carnivores nonetheless, which means they need a high amount of protein. Depending on the stage of life your furry friend is at, protein sources must be accompanied by a given portion of cereals and vegetables to make up for a balanced diet.

Let's say that you have a kitty and a senior cat in the same household. Although they are both house cats, kittens have a much higher energy demand, up to three times as much as an adult cat. In addition, about 1/3 of their energy comes straight from protein sources, which means that the proportion of protein in their meals should be higher for them to feel good. On the other hand, senior cats—and dogs—tend to have weaker joints, and they need higher amounts of calcium and collagen to stay strong and active.

And speaking of activity, what does a lifestyle full of activities that demand a lot of energy mean for your pet? More activity means that your pet's meals must meet a higher caloric intake that is also in agreement with its nutritional needs. For instance, let's go back to the cat example we used earlier, only this time with a second kitten. If two kittens from the exact same litter have a different routine, their nutritional requirements may look different. A cat that is very active, jumping around chasing things, playing, and all will obviously require much more energy than one that prefers to lie down in the sun for most of the day. Translating this scenario to see the bigger picture, in the case of carnivores more activity and younger age equal a higher demand for protein.

Although this is somewhat true for all animals, let's remember that every species is built with a different metabolism. For instance, even though cats get most of their energy from protein, dogs thrive on a diet that leans a bit more to the omnivore side—a direct consequence of their domestication—while herbivores like guinea pigs or rabbits rely on vegetables rich in complex carbohydrates and fiber. All foods are made up of different amounts of the exact same nutrients, and all animals need all types of nutrients as well. When selecting foods, the key lies in understanding how each type of nutrient works and the importance of the nutritional composition of food.

Understanding Nutrients

The first thing you need to know about nutrients is that, according to their chemical characteristics, they can be classified into two main groups: macronutrients and micronutrients. They were given these names based on how much of them are needed by the body, meaning that macronutrients—proteins, carbohydrates, and fats—must be ingested in large amounts, while micronutrients—mainly vitamins and minerals—come in much smaller quantities. To better understand the importance of each of these nutrients, we need to discuss what they are and how they work.

Protein

These molecules are arguably the most sought after by pet owners, especially because domestic animals that require high amounts of protein are very popular, particularly cats and dogs. A simple definition for proteins is that they are large molecules made up of amino acids. Proteins are crucial not only as a source of energy but also because they are the main component of muscles, which give your furry friend mobility and strength. In addition, proteins determine characteristics of the metabolic system and are also present in large quantities in hair, nails, and other body parts.

The body is perfectly capable of synthesizing the proteins that it needs to fulfill all of its requirements but to do so, it needs a good supply of building blocks: amino acids. These are attainable through the ingestion of high-quality protein, which means that in order to build strong and healthy muscles, your pet needs to synthesize protein through the assembly of amino acid chains, which come from yet another source of protein. Depending on your pet's species and breed, the source may be of animal or vegetable origin, and in some cases both. We'll talk more about where to get this nutrient from later in the book.

Carbohydrates

Commonly known as "carbs," these are molecules made up exclusively of carbon, oxygen, and hydrogen in particular arrays. They can be further categorized as sugars, starches, and fibers for nutritional purposes. Although there has been great debate about the role of carbohydrates in human and animal diets, we now know that they provide a very important immediate source of energy. Also, carbs take part in metabolic reactions that keep the body in a healthy state, contribute to a better digestive process, and adapt to energetic demands. Therefore, they should never be completely excluded from your pet's diet, even if they are not the main type of food for them.

Something important to remember about carbs is that you should always focus on providing your pet with complex carbohydrates rather than simple ones because they are a much healthier source of energy. You can find this type of carbs in all types of vegetables and unprocessed grains, which is yet another reason to turn to a homemade diet.

Fats

Fat is the name we commonly use for lipids, which are oily or greasy substances made up of carbon, oxygen, and hydrogen in specific arrangements. Along with carbs, fats have been heavily stigmatized and basically deemed as automatically unhealthy, but that couldn't be farther from the truth. To stay healthy, your pet definitely needs a small amount of fat, which will help with the absorption of micronutrients, while also serving as an energy storage, protection for organs, and regulator of body temperature.

This nutrient can also be subclassified according to certain chemical properties. First, we have unsaturated fats, which you may have heard of as "healthy fats," and are found in popular foods like olive oil, avocado, nuts, and fish. Healthy omega fats belong to this category, and they are known to help lower harmful LDL cholesterol, which contributes to good cardiovascular health for your pet. On the other hand, there are saturated fats, commonly known as "unhealthy fats," and are mostly found in highly processed foods and certain animal products like dairy and sausages. It is important to know that all foods contain both types of fats, and it is the proportion of them that changes, but worry not, I'll tell you more about how to include healthy fats in your pet's diet in later chapters.

Vitamins

As I told you at the beginning of the chapter, vitamins are micronutrients, which means they are substances needed in small amounts to perform most bodily functions. Just like it happens in humans, pets can produce some vitamins, but they need to get others through food. In order to provide your furry friend with its necessary vitamin intake, it is important that you know about some principles regarding the nature of vitamins.

First off, vitamins can be subdivided into two groups: fat-soluble and water-soluble. Vitamins A, D, E, and K belong to the first group, which means that they can be found in foods with high healthy fats content, like meat, eggs, nuts, seeds, and high-quality vegetable oils such as olive oil. Fat-soluble vitamins can be stored in your pet's organs, and they are also more resistant to temperature. Then we have vitamins C and B, which belong in the water-soluble group and cannot be stored in the body, they are rapidly absorbed and easily drained from their source when exposed to high cooking temperatures. Some of the best foods to provide your pet with these vitamins are raw fruits and vegetables, as well as broths and stocks, preferably obtained from low-heat cooking.

Minerals

Last but not least, we have another type of micronutrient, which are minerals. These are inorganic elements—mostly metals—that help in many metabolic processes. Just like us, our pets need a minimum intake of minerals like calcium, potassium, and sodium, and smaller amounts of trace minerals like zinc, copper, or iodine. Technically speaking, minerals come from soil and water, but because of the food chain, they end up in plants and products of animal origin such as milk and meat. During certain stages of life, it may be necessary to consider supplementation to fulfill the requirements, which is why your senior pet may need, for example, some extra calcium to help with its bones. Fortunately, a balanced diet and some natural alternatives are a great solution, but I'll tell you more about that later.

Balance and Portion Control

It is only logical to think about the importance of keeping good control over the portions of food we give to our pets, especially since many domestic animals are prone to eating as much as they possibly can, which can cause weight problems. On the other extreme of the spectrum, we have the picky eaters, with whom owners are likely to struggle to reach the minimum recommended nutrient intake. It is crucial that both of these problems are solved because balance and appropriate portions are key to good nutrition.

Depending on the type of pet you own, there are some approximations that may serve as a guide to start calculating the right portion. However, remember to always consider your pet's lifestyle, breed, and age to adjust the portions to its requirements, and always go to your vet if you notice anything strange about the amount of food your pet eats.

In the case of cats and dogs, there is a simple rule you can start by, which says that adult pets' meals are equivalent to about two to three percent of their weight, roughly 16 ounces of food for every 50 pounds in dogs and about four ounces per every 10 ounces for cats. For rodents, birds, and other small animals, there's less available information regarding the specific amount of food they need, but luckily they are pretty good at rationing food, so you could prepare their meals in batches and just administer it to fit their demand. Remember that, regardless of the pet you own, the best parameter to know if they are getting a good amount of food is their general health, particularly when it comes to weight. Because of this, it is crucial for them that you make sure they are in their optimal weight range, and they are active and alert, just doing whatever activities are normal for their breed and age without any trouble.

Chapter 2:

Safe and Nutritious Ingredients

Sharing delicious food we enjoy with our furry friends is an amazing way to bond, but it is very important that we are aware of what they can eat and what may be harmful to them. It is definitely a pity that our pets don't get to enjoy everything we consider a tasty treat, but that doesn't mean that they can't have delicious food. Lucky for us, every day it becomes easier to learn about ways to nourish our pets, create new recipes and avoid including foods that are good for us, but not for them. In this chapter, I'll tell you about ingredients that are considered safe for your pet and those that aren't, which will allow you to know how to create amazing meals for your beloved animal without putting them at any sort of risk.

Pet-Friendly Ingredients You Can Use

Unsurprisingly, there are lots of ingredients that are safe for your pets to eat. Of course, it is important to emphasize that this depends on the pet species, as there are some domestic animals that can eat almost the same things we do, while others need a very different set of ingredients. Another possibility worth considering is allergies because just like us, our pets can also be allergic to certain ingredients that are considered safe for them. To start with this list, we can mention foods that are safe for dogs and cats—the most common domestic animals—presenting them according to the type of food they belong to.

Safe Foods for Dogs and Cats

- *Protein sources.* Almost all types of meat work well in a dog's diet, but if you really want to step up your game, I would recommend beef, chicken, skinless salmon, and tuna. Bacon may also be a good option, with the only condition that it is completely natural and uncured. Chicken and cow liver are a favorite among dogs as well, and you can also add eggs as an amazing way to use something other than meat.

- *Carbohydrate sources.* Dogs and cats can get their carbs from some grains like whole-wheat flour—preferably gluten-free—rice flour, oats, carrot, and sweet potato. These foods not only provide them with sugars but also with high amounts of fiber to help with their digestion. Fruits and vegetables are also great to add some nice carbs to your pet's meals. Great options are apples, bananas, blueberries, cauliflower, mangoes, pears, peas, pumpkin, spinach, and watermelon. In addition to providing sugar and fiber, veggies are fantastic sources of vitamins and minerals, so be sure to find out some that your pet really enjoys and make them a part of every meal.

- *Fat sources.* Small amounts of high-quality vegetable oil are great choices to add to your pet's diet. Olive, sunflower, or coconut oil are the main oils that you should use to prepare their meals with, plus you can add small amounts of lactose-free dairy as another good source of healthy fats. Some seeds, also in small amounts, are also beneficial to provide your dog with the fats it needs; examples include chia, linseed, or peanuts.

Safe Foods for Other Small Mammals

If your furry friend is even tinier, chances are its diet will be different from that used for dogs and cats. However, small mammals—such as rodents—share a very similar diet with each other, regardless of their species. In fact, you may have heard that rodents will regularly eat just about anything we consider edible, but that doesn't mean all of those foods provide them with the right nutrition for them to thrive. As usual, remember that the meals and portions presented here are meant to serve as a base and should be adapted to your pet's needs. Now let's talk about some great ingredients you can use for their meals.

- *Protein sources.* Rodents are not that big on protein and domestic ones hardly ever consume meat, but they still need some foods rich in protein to stay healthy. You can provide them with these nutrients through unsweetened plain or low-sugar yogurt, chicken meat, and bones, unsalted nuts, or grains that are high in protein, such as oats.

- *Carbohydrate sources.* This is arguably the nutrient that small mammals need most, as it is their primary source of energy, so it makes sense that there are plenty of options to choose from. You can use most fruits and vegetables for their mix, including carrots, broccoli, cucumber, peas, pumpkin, green beans, bananas, apples, berries, kiwi, apples, or peaches. I would recommend the base to be made up of a variety of grains, like corn, barley, oats, rice, and even pasta or low-sugar low-sodium cereals made from these same grains.

- Fat sources. As you may have noticed, several of the foods I mentioned earlier are also amazing sources of healthy fats, particularly nuts, and yogurt, so you can just stick to that, since these little fellas don't really need that much of their diet to have fat in it.

Herbs, Condiments, or Spices For Your Pet

While most spices—and a considerable amount of herbs—are not considered safe for pets, there are some you can use. Not only will they help you create more flavorful meals, but your pet may also get great benefits from them. Just like some other ingredients, herbs can be used to prepare delicious meals and snacks to give some variety to your furry friend's menu.

Among the herbs you can use, there are cilantro leaves, dill tea, ginger, mint leaves, oregano, parsley, peppermint, rosemary, sage, and turmeric. You can add a little bit of black pepper or cinnamon as well, always using very small amounts. And make sure your pet doesn't sniff the powder directly, as it could be irritating for their eyes and airways. Chamomile is another option for dogs, but never use it for cats, since they are extremely sensitive to it.

As a bit of a disclaimer, remember that some herbs and spices are prone to triggering allergic reactions, so be sure to keep an eye on your pet when you try new ones, just in case. The amount of herbs you can use for your pet's meal should always be very small, normally ranging from ⅛ to ¼ of a spoon, depending on the herb. Also, keep in mind that although some of these herbs can be powdered or prepared as tea, essential oils are strictly forbidden, even if they come from the same plant, due to the fact that their chemical composition is toxic for most domestic animals' consumption.

Potentially Harmful Ingredients

As I said before, it is extremely important for your pet's well-being that you are always conscious about the foods that could harm them. There are always certain foods that we consider edible but may be poisonous for our pets, while others may trigger unpleasant side effects when eaten in bigger amounts. In addition, keep in mind that some pets could have allergic reactions to certain foods that would otherwise be safe for them. For these reasons, you should always watch out for signs of discomfort in your pet, like swelling, difficulty breathing, a notorious change in their poop, and belly pain, among others. Lucky for us, there is plenty of information about this, so it is not that hard to know what foods you should avoid.

Foods You Should Not Give to Your Dog

There are several foods that are known to be toxic to domestic animals like dogs or cats, so here I hand you a list of common human foods that you must avoid giving to your pet at all costs. Condiments like onion, garlic, mustard seeds, salt, and chives are dangerous for dogs, so never prepare their food with any of them. However, that doesn't mean you can't use any spices for your pet's food; just head back to the section about herbs and condiments earlier in this chapter, which you can use to make your pet's meal delicious, and provide other benefits. But more on that in the next section, let's get back to what you should not put on their plate.

Foods and beverages that tend to alter the heartbeat rhythm, like chocolate, alcohol, energy drinks, flavored drinks coffee, or tea—that contain caffeine—should also be avoided, as they can put your pet in danger. In fact, it is best for candy, in general, to be excluded from your pet's diet, as they have no nutritional value and, because they are highly processed and sugary, they could hurt your pet, be toxic, or cause allergies. Gum is also particularly dangerous because it can block your pet's throat, stomach, or gut. Additionally, sweet and processed foods that are labeled sugar-free often have artificial sweeteners instead, and some of those—like xylitol—are very toxic for pets. Bread that is made with yeast is not a good call either, so try to keep that away from your pet.

There are also some fruits and other veggies that pets shouldn't eat. For example, never give them grapes, avocado, corn cob, rhubarb, mushrooms—along with anything that contains mold—or any type of raisin. In the case of tomatoes, the leaves and stems should not be used to prepare their meals, while seeds or pits of fruits that are safe for pets should be avoided as well; such is the case of cherries, peaches, or apples. Certain nuts are not suitable for your pet's diet either, like walnuts and macadamia nuts. In addition, although you already know that protein of animal origin is the main ingredient for your pet's meals, avoid cooked bones at all costs, since they are likely to cause internal injuries and blockages. In the case of cats, also avoid all dairy, coconut-based products, of which dogs can only take small amounts of oil.

On a side note, raw animal protein is a great option for your pet, but there is always a chance that they may get an infection. Since they would be getting essentially the same benefits from a properly cooked protein, you can spare yourself the trouble and avoid raw chicken, beef, or fish altogether.

Foods You Should Not Give to Other Small Mammals

Some foods that we know and love are an absolute no-no when it comes to feeding small mammals, like rodents. For instance, despite them being able to eat most vegetables, they should definitely stay away from raw onion, celery, radishes, collards, beets, turnips, and avocados. As far as fruit goes, the only forbidden ones are citrus, although eating too many berries may cause them to have mild stomach aches and even diarrhea, so you don't have to avoid those, but do feed them a small amount. Other than that, just be careful about seeds, particularly apple seeds, which are highly poisonous for most animals. For other non-mammalian domestic animals, such as birds and reptiles, you can go with the same rules, with one additional detail: don't feed them fat. In the case of ferrets, be also aware of chocolate, which can cause severe intoxication and even death.

These lists are pretty good, but I urge all owners to double-check every ingredient they are having doubts about that was not included here. The reason is that, though here I considered the most common restrictions, it is always better to be sure if you decide to go for something that was not mentioned. Your pet's safety should always be your priority.

Where to Get Your Ingredients

As you can see, ingredients to make amazing meals for your pet are not unusual or hard to get at all. In fact, you may be able to get them conveniently at your favorite grocery store, but my personal recommendation will always be to get ingredients that are as fresh as possible, and what better way to do that than supporting your local producers.

If you want to give your furry friend some non-GMO ingredients that were obtained through environmentally responsible procedures, go to your local farmer's market. That way you'll ensure that these were carefully harvested, plus you can approach the producers personally and ask them about any doubts you have. Some products also come with tags that indicate whether they are organic or not, among other important features.

When you make your pet's meals with these fantastic ingredients, you're more likely to ensure that they are not consuming any toxic pesticides and that they get all of their nutrients with an amazing taste. There is honestly nothing better than that!

Chapter 3:

Kitchen Techniques and Tips

Things are definitely going to get more interesting in this chapter. I'm sure you know that when we make our own meals, every type of food needs to be prepared in a precise way to make sure that you get the most out of it. Well, the same thing goes for our pets! Remember that, to a certain level, making a balanced meal for our little ones involves mimicking the nutrients that they should be able to find in nature, and that often differs from the way we prepare our own meals. From measuring portions to cooking for the right amount of time, there are certainly a couple of techniques that you'll have to familiarize yourself with. In this chapter, I'm going to walk you through every step you have to follow to get the best recipes, from the gadgets that will make the process easier to how you should cook each type of food. That being said, let's start by gathering your essentials so you're ready to have some fun in the kitchen with your furry friend.

Tools and Equipment for Preparing Homemade Pet Meals

First things first: to know what you'll be using; you need to have an idea of what ingredients you'll be using most. For instance, if you're cooking for a dog or a cat, there will be a lot of protein, so you'll need things like good knives and designated chopping boards. On the other hand, if you're feeding birds or small rodents you may need hooks and food dispensers. See where we're going with this? It is obvious that every owner learns through practice what the best gadgets are, but having a nice list that covers all the basics will definitely help you build the perfect set.

Regardless of the type of pet you own, certain tools and equipment are equally useful. For example, whether you have a hamster or a dog, you'll need some good food storage containers. You can choose glass or plastic ones, just make sure that whichever material they are made of, it is important to check if they are microwavable and freezable. If you decide to batch-cook, you may be able to dedicate less time to cooking and be prepared all week, or even longer. Having your pet's portions always ready to heat up is a great way to save time, money, and energy!

Even if meal prepping is not your drill, having some high-quality containers is still important, as it will allow you to store ingredients the best way possible, making it easier to prepare them and even helping them last fresh for longer.

Yet another indispensable piece of equipment is a scale, along with a set of measuring spoons and cups. These will help you feed your pet with the right portions of food every single day. Once you grab a hold of it, weighing and measuring will become so much easier, and it will help you provide your pet with all of the benefits of an amazing natural meal.

A big and sturdy cutting board will also be helpful almost for any type of pet meal, but it is particularly useful if you'll be using lots of veggies like carrots, ginger, and others of the sort. If your pet is a big meat eater, make sure to designate a specific cutting board just for meat. This is crucial because cutting veggies or fruits on the same board you manipulate meat on increases the chances of getting cross-contamination, which is a huge risk factor for gastrointestinal infections. There are a variety of cutting boards you can choose from, but sturdy wood boards are most recommended, as they last a long time and are easy to work with.

Now continuing with the food for carnivore mammals, like cats or dogs, tools and bowls made of resistant materials are very important. Our pets can get naughty sometimes, so getting plates that aren't easy for them to move around or break will be a great help for you. Two great options include ceramic and stainless steel. If you have a small pet, ceramic bowls at ground level work fantastic, they are easy to clean, look good and they are heavy enough to stay in place. On the other hand, if you have a bigger pet—or an extremely active one that likes to move its plate around—stainless steel is a better option; these bowls are practically unbreakable, they are also easy to clean, and will stay with you for a long time. If your pet is more on the big side, you should also consider buying an additional piece that supports the bowl to elevate and make it more accessible for your pet, which will help prevent future neck issues.

Good quality knives and scissors are also a must. Remember that you'll be chopping different types of ingredients, like veggies and raw meat, so owning a couple of knives is really important. If possible, consider getting a full set of stainless steel knives, making sure you gather bread knives—which work amazing for tough meat—and carving knives for softer meat and viscera. Scissors will be your best friends when it comes to ingredients with a spongy consistency, and you can also try and find which knives work best for the veggies you add to their plate.

Last but not least: the fridge and cupboards. It may not look like it now, but ingredients and meals for your pet can take up a lot of space. Just think about all the space you use to store ingredients for your meals in the kitchen! Your pet will need a designated space for its food, whether you're meal-prepping or not. If you're planning on storing full portions—i.e., 15 days' worth of food—or some big stock of ingredients—like bone broth or other preparations—be sure you make some space in the freezer. Similarly, you may need to assign a specific space in your fridge for all the veggies, fruits, and so on. On the other hand, if you're including or basing your pet's diet on grains and seeds, make sure you can store them in a cool and dry space of your cupboards, preferably on hermetic containers. Now time to learn how to use all of these gadgets to make your pet some delicious meals.

Tips for Meal Prepping, Planning, Ingredient Preparation, and Storage

I'm sure you have already gotten some ideas as I introduced tools and gadgets for you, so in this section, we're ready to dive into some hacks you can use to make the whole process easier and more effective. At the end of the day, meal prepping for your pet shouldn't take up your whole life, it is just another activity that you'll get to share with them and hopefully enjoy doing, so here we go.

Meal-Prep for Pets

With its rising popularity, I'm sure most of us are a little bit familiar with the concept of meal-prep, but if that is not the case, I'll explain it in a very general way right here. Meal prep is a cooking technique that consists in preparing full dishes or key elements in advance, with the goal of saving time and money while creating delicious and nourishing meals. For example, if you plan on feeding your cat a tasty dish made up of fish, rice, and veggies, you have a couple of options for meal prep. You can either cook the ingredients and store them separately, by preparing big batches of foods divided by categories—i.e., Carbohydrates, protein, and complements—or ensemble full meals and storing each serving in a single recipient.

Whether you choose one option or the other fully depends on how comfortable you feel and what works best for your pets. There are a couple of tips I can give you though. For example, if your pet is a picky eater, they may enjoy their foods better when the flavors are fused together, or maybe they enjoy veggies crunchier, or soggier. It is these types of details that may help you determine the method that will work better for you.

In terms of functionality, you could also consider how much available time you have. For instance, if you have a day off that you can dedicate to meal prepping for your pet, it may be more efficient to spend a single day out of the whole week buying, cooking, storing, and organizing everything your pet will eat during the next seven days. Or maybe you can't afford to spend an entire day doing this, but you can dedicate 30 minutes a day, every afternoon, and that helps you prepare your pet's meal for the next day. Perhaps you're kind of in between; then you could prepare some nice bases for the week and then just assemble different dishes right before feeding your pet. As I said, it really all depends on what works best for you and your furry friend. I'd say that, in general, the best advice is to analyze all of the options and go for the one that you find easier. Then you'll find ways to improve it on the go until you create the perfect routine for you.

Remember that you can use meal prep for all types of pets and meals. If you own a small mammal, like a hamster or a rabbit, chances are you won't be cooking that much, but you could still prepare and store portions that contain the right combination of ingredients for an awesome meal. It may not look like much, but I promise it will be much easier to just grab a portion that is ready to be put on the plate instead of going through the trouble of looking for all of the ingredients every single time.

Meal Planning

Put into simpler words, meal planning is just a fancy way of saying that you'll create a menu for your pet, but we can give it a deeper meaning. When you plan a meal, not only are you taking care of making delicious recipes, but also making sure these dishes meet the nutritional requirements they are intended to.

Planning a meal involves portion sizes, supplementation, meal prepping, and much more, and should be done carefully if you want your pet to get all of the benefits its diet offers. As I have been saying, every animal is different, and you should always keep your mind open to adjust the diet to its requirements, but creating a structured plan makes it a lot easier.

First and foremost, you should calculate appropriate portions for your pet, taking into consideration its breed, age, and lifestyle. Once you have that, think about their nutritional requirements and their sources, from which you'll select the ingredients you will work with throughout the time you're planning the menu for. Once you're sure you have got everything you need, create a schedule that suits your pet's routine, and try to respect it as much as possible. As you continue to repeat this pattern, both you and your fur baby will engage with this new lifestyle and it will certainly become easier to sustain, and even add some variety to make things more exciting.

Ingredient Preparation

We can consider this a sibling of meal prep, as it involves planning ahead and leaving your ingredients ready to work with, the only difference is that this starts before all of that. To prepare your ingredients, you must first have a meal plan, which will allow you to know what ingredients to purchase. Once those ingredients make it home, you have to make sure that they are safe to use for your pet's meal, which means that you'll have to classify them, wash them, and maybe store them. Then, you can choose from several cooking techniques which will serve best to prepare them; I'll tell you more about that in the next section.

Storage

Proper meal storage has two goals: preserving the meals freshly and making the process easier for you. Remember that food is somewhat delicate, and you should avoid all risks of expiration and contamination. Making sure that your pet's meals, bases, and ingredients are safely stored will help you prevent gastrointestinal issues and infections, plus it will save you a lot of time.

How do you make sure you're storing everything properly? Simple, just think about what each type of food requires. Meats, fruits, vegetables, and cooked grains and cereals should always be refrigerated, and preferably stored in closed containers. If a cooked meal or raw piece of meat will require storage for a longer time—meaning over one week—consider freezing it to reduce the risk of dangerous microorganisms growing on it. Meanwhile, seeds, uncooked grains, oils, nuts, and some veggies can be stored in cool and dry spaces, preferably away from direct sunlight. When it comes to snacks, like baked goods and such, take into consideration the ingredients it has and whether they will last a long time before your pet eats them or not; this will indicate if it needs to be refrigerated or if they can stay at room temperature without further issues. If you're using raw veggies as a full snack, you can also use some specific techniques for them, like cutting them and putting them into a recipient with water. This tip works wonders to keep carrots fresh and crunchy.

Cooking Techniques

Back when I told you about the properties of each type of nutrient, you learned that certain compounds can only tolerate so much heat or are metabolized in a different way from one another. Well, here's how you're going to make sure that your pet gets the best out of every ingredient.

Almost as a general rule, animals thrive on food that is not overcooked, so keep in mind that on many occasions, you'll feed your pet meals that were prepared using different—or quicker—methods than what you would do for your own food. For example, to provide carnivores with the amount of protein they need, you have to make sure that the meat is just barely cooked, as the only goal here is to prevent any possible infection while preserving the meat's natural properties and consistency as possible. In the case of veggies, which are a great source of micronutrients, do not waste the broth and always cook them at low heat.

If you're wondering how you can achieve the right level of cooking, there are some famous techniques that will become your best friends. Processes like steaming work wonders when it comes to veggies, as it allows them to preserve their soluble vitamin content while making them easier to eat and digest for your pets. Baking is also a good technique, and it can be used for all sorts of foods. Preparations that include grains, meat, and veggies can be baked to get that juicy finish, plus it allows you to cook larger amounts of food, and many times the results are freezer-friendly. In case you prefer to cook your pet's food in a simpler or more traditional way, you can opt for slow cooking, which means that you can prepare meals using low heat for as long as needed. For example, if you would normally cook carrots for 20 minutes at medium temperature, your furry friend may benefit more from having them cooked at low heat for half an hour. Remember that choosing one of these techniques does not mean you can't get experimental with the rest of them, so have some fun making different foods and using various techniques!

Chapter 4:

Tail-Wagging Recipes for Dogs

Are you ready to dive into the fun world of dog recipes? If so, you have reached the core of the book and what probably brought you here in the first place. If you have a dog at home, chances are that they have stared at you while you're having dinner with those bright puppy eyes asking you to share some of it with them. Sadly, as you read said earlier, many of the foods we love are not safe for our furry friends, which means that sharing our meals with them is not a great call. However, that doesn't mean we can make them something that they enjoy just as much and that nourishes them the way they deserve.

In this chapter, we're going to see some recipes that are specially designed for dogs at certain stages of life. You'll also get a couple of ideas for dogs living with specific health conditions, all of which are prepared with ingredients that are recommended for your dog's case. If you happen to like one of the recipes presented here but feel like they require further modifications due to their lifestyle, physical activity, picky eating, or health condition, feel free to follow the tips and ingredients that were included in other chapters to create your own perfect version of these meals. Now let's get right into it.

Delicious and Nourishing Recipes for Your Dog

All of the following recipes are vet approved but keep in mind that every dog is different, and although these dishes are tailored for dogs, you may need to adjust ingredients and portions. The meals presented here are meant to serve as a guide for you to start giving your pup some nutritious and delicious homemade meals, enjoy!

Recipes for Puppies

Earlier in the book, I talked about how puppies tend to have a relatively large need for protein, or at least more than adult dogs do. In general, they may also need food that is gentle on their stomach and tastes amazing. During this stage of a dog's life, it is also easier to introduce them to new flavors and textures, which is an amazing investment for their later years, as it will allow them to have a much more varied diet and you will have many more options to choose from. Time to start with some simple dishes that every puppy will love.

Chicken and Spinach Meal

- Ingredients. Gather 1 ½ cups of brown rice—this one is better for your dog's digestion– along with 4 pounds of ground chicken, 4 cups of spinach leaves, 15 ounces of tomato sauce, 2 yams, and a tablespoon of olive oil. Remember that if you want to make smaller or bigger batches, you can just adjust the amounts of ingredients while respecting the proportions of them.

- Preparation.

    a. Cook the rice, using nothing else but water. Pre-cooked rice regularly takes about 10 minutes, and raw rice will take around 20 minutes.

    b. Simultaneously cook the yams until tender, using the microwave, an air fryer, or boiling it. Don't forget to pierce some holes in it first, and rotate it halfway through the time so it cooks evenly. Once it's done, cut it into smaller pieces.

    c. Cook the chicken along with the olive oil on medium heat.

    d. Remove the chicken pot from the heat and add the cooked rice and yams, along with the tomato sauce and spinach. Mix together and then blend it until you get a homogenous mixture.

e.   Let it cool and line it on trays or plates. Now you can scoop and serve it to your pup or store individual portions in the freezer.

Turkey and Veggie Dish

- Ingredients. Get 3 pounds of turkey—preferably ground—1 ½ cups of brown rice, 3 cups of spinach, 2 carrots, 1 zucchini, ½ cups of peas, and a tablespoon of olive oil. Again, you can adjust the amounts so you can meal prep or make smaller portions.

- Preparation.

    a.   Cook the brown rice—you can use the instructions on the previous recipe—and meanwhile it's ready, shred the carrots and zucchini, and chop the spinach leaves.

    b.   Separately cook the turkey until it turns brown— normally about 5 minutes is enough—and then add the cooked rice along with the vegetables.

    c.   Stir to mix and cook everything together for another 5 minutes.

    d.   Let the meal cool down and serve it to your puppy or store individual portions for later.

Recipes for Senior Dogs

Because senior dogs have some similar nutritional requirements as puppies, you might notice that dishes don't look different. Nonetheless, they often need meals that are gentler on their stomach, easier to chew, and that helps their digestion. Here I'll present you with two recipes that will work wonders on your senior buddy.

Beef and Veggie Stew

- Ingredients. You will need a pound of beef stew meat, ½ cup of green beans, ½ cup of carrot, a sweet potato, ½ cup of flour, a tablespoon of olive oil, and ½ cup of water. Carrots and green beans must be diced.

- Preparation.

    a. Cook the sweet potato until tender but somewhat firm—you can use the techniques mentioned in the first puppy recipe.

    b. Heat up the olive oil and add small chunks of the meat—about the size of a coin—and then let it cook until well done, for about 15 minutes.

    c. Take the meat out and make a thick gravy in the same pan by adding water and flour, then whisk until you get a thick and homogeneous consistency.

    d. In the same pan, add the rest of the ingredients and mix until the gravy covers everything up. Cook on low heat for 10 minutes, until everything is tender.

    e. Let the meal cool down and serve or store it.

Turkey and Veggie Rice Bowl

- Ingredients. Get 2 cups of brown rice, two cups of chopped broccoli, carrot, and cauliflower mixture, a pound of ground turkey, a tablespoon of dried rosemary and 6 cups of water.

- Preparation.

    a. Cook the vegetables for about 5 minutes, and remove them from the heat just as they start to get a little tender. Reserve.

b. Heat up the water, and once it reaches a boil, add the rice, turkey, and rosemary. Make sure to stir and break down the turkey clumps. Let the mixture simmer for about 20 minutes on low heat.

c. Add the veggies and cook for another 5 minutes.

d. Remove the mixture from the heat and let it cool down completely before serving or storing.

Recipes for Adult Dogs and Options for All Ages

The recipes I will share with you in this section are safe for all ages and breeds but are particularly suitable for adult dogs. Here, you will also find some other protein options you can incorporate into their diet. Ready for it?

Egg and Beef Rice Bowl

- Ingredients. You will need 2 pounds of ground beef, 4 eggs, 6 cups of rice, 3 carrots, 3 tablespoons of olive oil, and ¼ cup of curly parsley.

- Preparation.

    a. Heat up some water and bring it to a boil. Then put in the eggs for about 8 to 10 minutes or until fully cooked. A pro tip to peel them is to transfer them into cool water, and then peel carefully and chop them up.

    b. Cook the ground beef until brown with the olive oil.

    c. Cook the brown rice using just water.

    d. Meanwhile, shred the carrots and chop the parsley. Reserve.

e. Now mix all of those ingredients together, and let them simmer for about 5 minutes, including the carrots and rice.

f. Wait until the meal cools down completely, then serve or store for later.

Fish and Veggie Meal

- Ingredients. Gather 1 ½ cups of brown rice or oatmeal, 2 pounds of white fish of your preference, a can of salmon or tuna, 3 eggs, and 3 cups of diced veggies of your choice—you can go for carrots, broccoli, and zucchini.

- Preparation.

    a. Start by cooking the fish for about 5 minutes, and then chop or grind it into smaller pieces.

    b. Cook your rice or oatmeal, and while that is ready, bring another pot of water to a boil and add the veggies in for about 5 to 10 minutes.

    c. Boil your eggs and then peel them and chop them into smaller pieces—you can use the tip I gave you in the last recipe to peel them faster.

    d. Combine all of the ingredients and mix them really well, then allow them to cool down and serve to your pet or store in the freezer for later.

Meal Ideas for Dogs Living With Specific Health Conditions

Recently, veterinary experts and many pet owners have been claiming that a homemade diet is the way to go when it comes to dogs living with chronic health conditions. In Chapter 6 you will learn about certain ground rules that may be useful to create balanced meals to help your dog thrive in spite of their diagnosis, but for now, I will leave here a few ideas you can take as a guide to create meals that suit your dog's needs. Again, feel free to take the inspiration and switch up some ingredients to create variations for your furry friend's menu.

Sweet Beef Pumpkin Bowl for Dogs With Kidney Disease

- Ingredients. You'll need 2 pounds of lean ground beef, a cup of egg whites, 2 cups of brown rice, 1 pound of green beans, 1 sweet potato, 2 cups of pumpkin, 1 apple, ½ cup of dried parsley, and 2 tablespoons of coconut oil.

- Preparation.

  a. First cook the ground beef until brown, along with the chopped green beans and sliced sweet potato.

  b. In a separate pan, heat up the coconut oil and fry the egg whites until fully cooked in the form of an omelet.

  c. Cook the rice according to the package's instructions and reserve.

  d. Boil the pumpkin until tender, and keep the fleshy part of it. If you're using canned pumpkin puree, make sure that is the only ingredient. In the same pot, mix together the pumpkin puree, the parsley, and the cooked egg whites. Reserve.

  e. In the blender or food processor, mash together ⅔ of the cooked ground beef mixture.

  f. Finally, in a big bowl, transfer the cooked rice and add the pureed mixtures from the previous steps. Then add the leftover whole ground beef mixture and stir until fully incorporated. Let it cool down completely and serve it to your dog or store it for later.

Chicken and Veggie Bowl for Dogs With Diabetes

- Ingredients. You will need 2 chicken breasts, 2 cups of brown rice, a cup of chopped asparagus, a cup of broccoli, and a teaspoon of parsley.

- Preparation.

  a. First, boil the skinless chicken breasts using only water. Once fully cooked, take out the chicken breasts and wait for them to cool down.

  b. Using the chicken stock left in the pan, cook the brown rice—add more water if needed—for about 10 minutes.

  c. Then add the broccoli, asparagus, and parsley to the rice, and let it cook for another 10 to 15 minutes, until the veggies are tender but still a little firm.

  d. Once the chicken breasts have cooled down, cut them into little pieces and then add it to the rice and veggie mixture.

  e. Wait for the meal to cool down and then serve it to your dog or store it for later.

Superfoods and Supplementation

According to the American Kennel Club, some of the best supplementations for your dog include glucosamine—an amino acid that helps them keep healthy joints—salmon oil which is rich in omega-3 fatty acids, and probiotics. A balanced diet should be able to provide your dog with all of the nutrients it needs, but supplementation may be advised under certain circumstances or during older age. In any case, you can consult with your veterinary specialist to see when you should be supplementing your dog.

Chapter 5:

Feline Favorites: Recipes for Cats

Similarly to Chapter 4, here you'll be presented with some amazing recipes that you can prepare for your beloved cat. The goal is for you to get started into the wonderful routine of homemade meals for your pets, and use these recipes as a guide to create the optimal menu for your furry friend. As mentioned in the previous chapter, cats require specific nutrients depending on their age, lifestyle, and health conditions, so here you'll be provided with some options that are designed for different types of necessities. As always, feel free to head to other chapters in this book for guidance on how to swap ingredients and tips to create better meals for your cat if they live with a particular diagnosis.

Delicious and Nourishing Recipes for Your Cat

Just as mentioned in the previous chapter about dogs, cats require specific nutrients depending on their age, lifestyle, and health conditions, so here you'll get some options that are designed for different types of necessities. If needed, head to other chapters in this book for guidance on selecting the right ingredients to meet your cat's needs.

Recipes for Kittens

Tuna Balls

- Ingredients. Take 2 cans of tuna, 4 tablespoons of oat flour, 1 tablespoon of olive oil or butter, ½ cup of breadcrumbs, and an egg.

- Preparation.

    a. Preheat your oven to 325 °F and prepare a tray with parchment paper.

    b. Throw the breadcrumbs into a bowl and add the olive oil or melted butter, then mix that until you get lumps of breadcrumbs.

    c. Add the tuna, egg, and oat flour to the previous mixture and incorporate everything together.

    d. Make little balls out of the mixture—about ½ inch in size—and place them on the tray. Bake for about 10 minutes.

    e. Take them out and allow them to cool down. Now they're ready for your kitty to eat, or you can store them in the fridge for later.

Chicken Mix Bowl for Kittens

- Ingredients. Gather 50 grams of chicken liver, 100 grams of chicken heart, 700 grams of chicken wings, 100 grams of salmon, 50 grams of beef kidney, 1 egg, and ½ cup of rice.

- Preparation.

a.   Boil the meat ingredients until tender using 2 cups of water, being really careful not to let it overcook. This will take about 15 to 20 minutes.

b.   Throw the mixture in a meat grinder or high-powered blender. Make sure to leave bones out, since cooked bones are dangerous for your pet's digestive tract.

c.   Cook the rice according to the package's instructions, which is normally about 10 to 20 minutes.

d.   Mix everything together and add the powdered egg shells and some raw bones on top of the mixture for some extra calcium. Wait for everything to cool down and serve it to your cat or store for later.

Recipes for Senior Cats

Chicken and Tuna Meal for Senior Cats

- Ingredients. ½ of cooked vegetables of your choice—I recommend zucchini, broccoli, and carrot—, a chicken breast, a can of tuna, and 2 tablespoons of olive oil.

- Preparation.

  a.   Cook the skinless and boneless chicken breast, then drain and shred it.

  b.   Add in the tuna.

  c.   Chop the vegetables into smaller pieces and bring to a boil for about 10 minutes or until tender.

  d.   Blend all of these ingredients together, then wait until it cools down and serve it to your cat or store it for later.

Beef and Rice Bowl

- Ingredients. Gather 1 ½ cups of ground beef, ½ cup of brown rice, ¾ cup of low-sodium cottage cheese, and ½ cup of alfalfa sprouts.

- Preparation.

    a. Cook the beef in a pan until brown and reserve.

    b. Bring the rice to a boil until fully cooked, which will take about 20 minutes.

    c. Chop the alfalfa sprouts into pieces as small as you can.

    d. Incorporate all of the ingredients together—also blend if you prefer—and let them cool down. Now the meal is ready for your cat, or you can store it for later.

Recipes for Adult Dogs and Options for All Ages

Chicken and Quinoa Bowl for Cats

- Ingredients. Get 2 skinless and boneless chicken breasts, 50 grams of quinoa, 2 to 3 cups of chopped spinach, and a tablespoon of olive oil.

- Preparation.

    a. Cook the chicken breasts by baking or boiling them, and then shred them completely.

    b. Bring the quinoa to a boil with a cup of water until the grains feel soft.

    c. Add the chopped spinach to the quinoa pot and remove from the heat. Incorporate by stirring until the spinach leaves wilt down.

    d. Add the shredded chicken into the pot and incorporate everything together once again.

e. Optional, you can use some of the leftover chicken broth to blend the mixture if your cat likes pate-like meals better. Let it cool down and serve it to your cat or store it for later.

Turkey and Squash Meal

- Ingredients. Get 100 grams of turkey breast, 150 grams of squash—or zucchini— 200 grams of spinach, and 2 tablespoons of olive oil.

- Preparation.

    a. Start by roasting the turkey breast and shredding it. You can also buy unseasoned low-sodium previously roasted turkey breast and skip directly to the shredding part.

    b. Take the squash to a boil and cook until tender but still firm, which will take 5 to 10 minutes. Add in the spinach and let it boil for another minute. Turn off the heat and drain the vegetables.

    c. Blend the ingredients together along with the olive oil until you get a paste-like texture.

    d. Allow the mixture to cool down and serve it to your cat or store it for later.

Meal Ideas for Cats Living With Specific Health Conditions

Chicken and Veggie Meal for Cats With Kidney Disease

- Ingredients. ½ cup of chopped green beans, ½ cup of shredded carrot, ½ cup of skinless and boneless chicken breast, ½ cup of rice, 2 eggs, a few drops of fish oil, and a tablespoon of olive oil.

- Preparation.

    a. Bake or boil the chicken breast until fully cooked, shred, and reserve.

    b. Cook the vegetables together until tender. Reserve.

    c. Bring the rice to a boil with 2 cups of water, then let it cook for about 20 minutes.

    d. Cook the egg on low heat in a similar form to scrambled eggs. Remove from the heat once it's cooked but still soft.

    e. Mix all of the ingredients together and allow to cool down to serve to your cat or store for later.

Turkey Patties for Diabetic Cats

- Ingredients. Get a pound of ground turkey, 2 eggs, and a cup of veggies of your choice—you can go for old reliable zucchini and carrots.

- Preparation.

    a. Cook the turkey until brown on low heat.

    b. Bring the vegetables to a boil and cook them until tender.

    c. In a bowl, mix the cooked ingredients along with the raw eggs and incorporate everything together. You can also add crushed egg whites for some additional calcium.

    d. Cook the mixture for about 5 to 10 minutes in a pan on low heat, then allow it to cool down and cut it into small squares or circles for your cat to enjoy or store for later.

Superfoods and Supplementation

Although a balanced diet is the key to optimal nutrition, your cat may need additional supplementation, especially during certain stages of life. A taurine supplement is one of the best supplements you can include in your cat's food, as it is crucial for heart health and not too easy to get from food. Your cat may also benefit from L-lysine supplements, probiotics specially designed for cats and joint-health supplements—the latter are particularly important for seniors—and some mineral substitutes.

Chapter 6

Special Diets for Specific Health Conditions

Finding the optimal diet for a pet living with a health condition can be a real challenge, especially if you are looking for ways to go more naturally about it. More often than not, pet owners—particularly animals that are undergoing some type of medical treatment—are told to keep them on a strict diet consisting of boring prescription food. Cans of wet food, dry pellets, and treats that don't really have a good flavor and are fully artificial are the most common elements of said diets, but let's be honest: it doesn't sound as good as a delicious home-cooked meal. In this chapter, you're about to learn about the importance of diet regarding some common health problems in pets, along with some tips on how to create meals that help create a better lifestyle for your furry friend.

The Role of Nutrition in Health and Specific Health Conditions

While fortunately, many health problems in pets have effective treatments, not all diseases can actually be cured, so managing them is more about keeping them under control so that your little buddy has as good of a quality of life as possible. Commercial pet foods often contain ingredients that may trigger or worsen certain health problems, making it harder for pets and their owners.

Because managing health conditions properly has been proven to open the possibility for a longer life expectancy and a better quality of life, pet owners and their health specialists have shined a light on the role of diet when it comes to these cases. With the pet food industry coming up with so many options for special health conditions, it is only logical to inquire whether homemade food can fulfill the same role as commercial prescription diets do. Interestingly enough, recent information proves that pets can benefit from a proper homemade diet. The key is to prepare meals that suit all of your pet's needs so that their diet helps them feel better while eating delicious dishes. Up next, I will present to you a brief explanation of the role of diet in some specific health conditions, along with some recommendations you can follow to tailor the perfect menu for your pet to thrive.

Dietary Recommendations for Pets With Specific Conditions

Allergies

Dealing with allergies can get a little tricky because some of the symptoms that come with it often resemble those of other health issues. For example, allergens that come in commercial pet food, and are thus directly absorbed by the intestinal tract, may occasionally lead to symptoms like diarrhea, vomiting, or loss of appetite. As you can see, all of these are also signs of gastrointestinal infections and other illnesses, leading owners to believe that the actual problem can't have anything to do with allergies.

In other cases, symptoms are much more obvious, consisting of rashes, itchiness, shaking, or redness. Nonetheless, even in this case, many owners don't immediately think of food allergies, particularly when their pet has not had a history of these issues.

The thing is that there are several foods that can trigger your pet's immunological system and thus cause them to have an allergic reaction, and you don't even have to think as far as unusual ingredients. Some frequent allergens include beef, chicken, and wheat, while other less common ones are nuts, eggs, or soy.

Unfortunately, the only effective way to diagnose, prove and treat a pet allergy is through a process known as an elimination diet trial, which lasts about two or three months. During that time, the pet owner must remove all proteins that you find suspicious of causing your furry friend's allergy, preferably with the guidance of a veterinary expert. The goal is to give their little body enough time to actually detox from that allergen and go back to normal.

On a different note, there are of course other types of allergies that don't happen in the gastrointestinal tract. These are usually treated using specific drugs that aim at helping reduce unsettling symptoms like inflammation or rashes, but hardly ever target the actual cause of the allergy. In addition, most of these treatments are aggressive or create resistance, and thus should not be used for extensive time periods. So, is there anything to be done through a diet that helps fight this off? As a matter of fact, there is.

One of the most common types of allergies in pets—especially mammals—is skin allergy, which normally shows up as a series of symptoms that include loss of hair, irritation, redness, and continuous scratching. Eliminating additives and conservatives from commercial pet food is a great first step toward healthier skin and coat, but if you want to go beyond that, it is time to be a little bit extra and tailor a diet that gives your pet that extra boost they need.

My best suggestion if your pet struggles with skin allergy is to include in their meals a generous amount of foods that help support their immune system. This will help them reduce exaggerated immune reactions, and with a lot of patience and a little luck, it could even get them off meds. Some of the best foods to help you get there are those that have a high content of omega-3 fatty acids—commonly referred to as healthy fats—along with antioxidants, lots of soluble fiber, and lean protein. Examples of these foods include fish, turkey, flaxseed, pumpkin, sweet potatoes, or berries, among many others. Back in Chapters 4 and 5, I presented you with some amazing and tasty options that incorporate these foods into delicious meals. Feel free to go take a look at it if you are considering this type of diet for your pets!

Diabetes

Just like it happens with every other health condition, not all diabetic pets benefit from the exact same diet, nor do they all manifest all of the same symptoms. Diabetes is a multifactorial chronic-degenerative disease that affects the quality of life of those who live with it, including our furry friends. There is a strong genetic factor that puts our pets at risk of developing diabetes, but there is an even stronger influence that comes from environmental factors, such as their diet and physical activity.

Much like us, most pets can get Type 1 and Type 2 diabetes, but in their cases, it's much more frequent to be diagnosed with Type 1 diabetes, which is a condition where they are unable to produce insulin. Unfortunately, diabetes doesn't have a cure, but it can be effectively treated so that our pets enjoy a life that is as close to normal as possible.

Lucky for us, there are already medications designed to treat diabetes in pets. If your fur baby is experiencing symptoms of this disease, such as sudden weight loss, changes in appetite, cloudy eyes, excessive water drinking, or recurring skin and urinary infections, please go to your vet to get proper treatment. However, we're here to find solutions within food. Does it sound crazy? Well, not at all.

Lifestyle changes are incredibly important when it comes to having a better quality of life for your pet. In a way, we could say that, with an adequate diet tailored to their needs, food can help your pet feel its best and enjoy a happy active life in spite of diabetes.

There is no "diabetic diet" per se, as every pet is different and therefore requires a diet that meets all of its needs, taking into consideration their likes and dislikes. However, we can speak about the basics of nourishing a pet that lives with diabetes, starting with the nutritional balance that works best for most cases.

As with regular diets, we have to start by making sure that you include a minimum amount of certain nutrients, only in these cases do you have to be even more aware of not going over the limits. That is, you need to hit a minimum amount of carbohydrates for your pet with diabetes to thrive, but you also have to make sure that your pet doesn't go over an acceptable sugar limit.

Water and carbohydrates are the most important elements to consider when feeding a diabetic pet because they are the main nutrients that will help keep insulin at optimal levels. Among the carbohydrates, fiber, and sugars are the most relevant ones, as fiber helps the body better absorb glucose, ensuring an acceptable blood sugar level. In most cases, hitting a good amount of high-quality protein—meaning going well above the minimum recommended amount—is also key to controlling diabetes. Remember that protein helps with muscle building, which is one of the most effective ways to use up ingested sugar.

Although it may sound pretty obvious, there is no harm in remembering that avoiding certain foods altogether may be a good measure to take care of your pet if it lives with diabetes. For instance, you should stay away from sugary and starchy foods, like very sweet fruits, such as mangoes or bananas. If your pet is also struggling with other underlying conditions, like obesity or high blood pressure, cutting down on fats and sodium will be a great boost for them, and as a sort of side effect, it may help with diabetes as well.

Kidney Disease

"Your pet has kidney disease" are probably some of the scariest words pet owners could hear, but one thing to note is that many pets can enjoy a comfortable life when properly treated against this diagnosis. Currently, most medication indicated to treat kidney disease is meant to keep symptoms under control, and hardly any target the actual causes. However, there is something else that you can do for your pet, and that has been proven to help little guys with this disease double their life expectancy and get rid of most symptoms: feed them a customized diet that suits their health needs.

Yes, you read that right. According to Vet Nutrition's 2016 bulletin, pets that stick to diets designed especially for kidney disease can live up to two times longer than those who live with this diagnosis and only have a regular diet. Although like in most other chronic diseases every patient is different, there are certain ground rules you can follow for most cases. For instance, owners of pets with kidney disease are almost always advised to help them cut down on minerals like phosphorus and sodium, plus minimize protein. At the same time, they should be supplementing their pets with some extra omega-3 fatty acids, preferably obtained from fish and fish oil.

The goal of this diet is to prevent protein and metal buildup from happening in the kidneys since they are the organs in charge of processing the protein that comes from food. In the case of mineral reduction, it's particularly important because trouble processing them leads to high blood pressure, which fastens kidney damage. You can start this process by removing commercial treats and replacing them with healthy snacks, like your pet's favorite fruits and vegetables.

Some popular high protein treats, like meat bits, cheese, or jerky treats could be really damaging to your pet if they live with kidney disease, so as much as they try to convince you to get some of it, say no. If you also include commercial food in your pet's diet, particularly canned wet food, try your best to avoid it as they tend to be pretty high in sodium and somewhat caloric.

Another detail that may help your pet is switching to an alkaline diet. This is because kidney disease tends to produce more acidic byproducts, so you really will want to keep that pH at a good level. In case you're wondering what foods will help you get there, I have some examples for you. Some delicious and refreshing treats that are great for your furry friend include zucchini, cucumber, pumpkin, apple, blueberries, and watermelon. For protein and carbs sources, the simpler the better, so you can stick to turkey, white fish, lean beef meat, chicken, green beans, beets, and rice. Oats will also be an amazing ally for your pet, as they help fight off acidity and high blood pressure, which means a better prognosis for kidney disease symptoms.

Picky Eaters

Sure, this is not a disease on its own, but I think we can all agree that picky eating can be the start of other health issues. If your pet's behavior changes after a particular event that has them stressed out, like a medical intervention or moving to a different house, it's kind of understandable that there is some loss of appetite. More often than not, in these cases, that type of behavioral changes don't last long, and hardly ever affect your pet in the long term. However, if due to whatever circumstance the picky eating has lasted longer than a few days, your pet may be at risk of developing further health issues.

Pets that have a hard time meeting their nutritional needs tend to have lower levels of important nutrients, like iron or sugar. Over time, this lack of nutrients may turn into problems like anemia, loss of muscle mass, chronic fatigue, a weaker immune system, osteoporosis, and hairless skin patches.

Nonetheless, one of the many perks of homemade diets is the possibility to cater a menu that suits all of your pet's needs, including tasty food that they actually enjoy. Imagine that you have trouble eating your food because you don't like its texture or flavor... but that's the only thing you can eat. Wouldn't it be awful? A homemade diet will allow your pet to actually like what they're eating, and even truly look forward to it every day!

Okay, what can you do to make a diet that is picky eater friendly? Easy, you just need to focus on including foods that your pet absolutely loves. If you have a dog or a cat, one of the safest ways to go is chicken, but you can try different sources of protein that are tempting for your pet. Many picky eaters enjoy different presentations of ground beef, and prefer their veggies to stay hidden. You can also opt for using broths and stocks to give that delicious meaty taste to other foods, like rice, potato, or pumpkin.

The case of smaller animals is not too different, so for instance, you can try to find out what that special food is for your hamster, bird, or rabbit. Yes, unfortunately, there is no better way of finding it than through trial and error, so you will have to observe your little one pretty closely so you can narrow it down to its favorite ingredients. If you are lucky, you will find one of its favorite foods among the best components of their diet; so for instance, if your bird happens to love a particular type of seeds, you can just let those be the major part of the dish! On the other hand, if your cat seems to love rice but not chicken, you are in serious need to find another source of protein. Do you see where we're going here? With picky eaters, you will always have two priorities: to create a balanced meal and to convince your pet to eat it.

Are there general rules that apply to all picky eaters? Sadly, there are not, because when you know a picky eater you only know that one, they can all have their own likes and dislikes, and be very different from one another. But fortunately, there are a couple of tips that work for almost every pet. First, keep your ingredients simple, just gather the nutritional sources to meet their needs. Start by giving them the most basic meals and build up from there, later you can help them try small pieces of new ingredients with similar tastes or textures to the ones they already like. You can also try giving them friendlier presentations like baked treats or porridges, covering new foods in preparations made of their favorite ingredients like veggies inside a meatball, among other ideas. Remember, the goal is to help these little furry guys to get enough nutrients to thrive.

Chapter 7

Catering to Small Pets

Creating homemade meals for other small pets is a big challenge, as they often consume much more limited ingredients. For instance, maybe you have a hard time making a meal for a rodent because they're not big cooked food eaters. However, in this chapter, I will show you a few ingredient combinations you can use as a guide to preparing amazing homemade meals for your small pet. Here we go.

Specialized Diets and Recipes

Rabbits

Like all other animals, how much food you give to your rabbit will depend on its size, weight, age, and level of physical activity. For the average house rabbit, you can create a great bowl of food by mixing together anywhere from one to three cups of leafy greens with just a little bit of other vegetables and edible flowers. This should be enough for an entire day, along with unlimited hay or grass, which are always the base for a rabbit's proper nourishment. Fruit can also be included in smaller amounts, as it is too sugary to be given to rabbits on a regular basis.

Guinea Pigs

There are two key features to create the perfect meal for your guinea pig: freshness and crunchiness. Start by getting a variety of veggies that are safe for your little furry guy, like bell peppers, and red-leaf lettuces. Make a small bowl consisting mostly of leafy greens, and then just a little amount of sugary vegetables like carrots and snap peas. Other ingredients you can throw in are small pieces of cucumber, celery, and bell peppers, all of which are amazing sources of vitamins and very low in sugar.

For small mammals like guinea pigs, rabbits, or hamsters, you can also make easy, baked treats. Most of these consist simply of a pureed fruit of your choice that is safe for your pet, such as bananas, pear, or apple, mixed with oat flour or regular all-purpose flour. Once you have a paste-like consistency, you can just bake them for about 10 minutes on low heat and wait for them to cool down before giving them to your pet. However, keep in mind that you should only give them small amounts of these treats and it's best to use them sporadically.

Birds

It's no secret that birds' diets consist mainly of grains and seeds. Nonetheless, I think it's important to mention that there are some grains that don't do much for your bird, so you should avoid them as they're considered "filler grains". Unfortunately, many commercial mixes contain these filler grains like sorghum, which leads us to conclude that your pet bird would be much better off with a homemade mix.

A great homemade mix option for your bird consists of ½ cup of striped sunflower seeds, a cup of black oil sunflower seeds, ½ cup of cracked corn, two spoons of white millet, a cup of unsalted crushed peanuts, and ⅛ cup of dried fruits.

Chapter 8:

Treating and Training With

Healthy Snacks

All pets love to have a delicious treat, with no exceptions. Preparing homemade treats and snacks for your furry friend is most definitely one of the best ways to bond with them, and if you choose wisely, it may even help you compliment their diet. If you think that handing out treats often to your pet is unhealthy, you're not alone. The pet food industry offers a wide variety of treats that are highly processed, and hardly ever provide any nutritional value for pets.

Average treats for pets are made of low-quality ingredients and mostly contain refined carbohydrates, which do nothing for your pet's health. If you're lucky, you may be able to find a couple of treats that include somewhat better ingredients, like traces of bones, skin, or certain types of meat. Still, many—if not most—of these products tend to cause further health problems, like obesity, lack of energy, and tooth damage. Can the all-mighty homemade diet help reduce these risks? Sure. Let's see how.

Homemade treats are made of ingredients you have full control over, which means that they can be as nutritious as you want them to be. As opposed to the average store-bought treats, you can use high-quality ingredients that your pet loves and gets some amazing benefits from. If we're talking about a carnivore mammal, some popular ingredients for treats are peanut butter, banana, apple oats, or chicken liver. You can also use some herbs and spices to make them tastier and provide additional benefits, such as cinnamon, parsley, or coconut oil. These are rich in antioxidants, help prevent bad breath, and even have anti-inflammatory properties, which makes them amazing options.

How to Use Treats in Training

It is no secret that creating a positive association between a command and an action is the best way to get your pet to learn some new tricks. From funny tricks like a high five to very useful ones like having your pet sit quietly when you need them to, there's nothing that can't be achieved through patience and delicious treats. And if you can take advantage of that process to bond with your pet and nourish them, well that's the whole package right there.

To get there, start by prepping some tasty treats using ingredients you're certain your pet will love—I'll talk you through it step by step in the next section—and if possible get them to join you. Then create the association between the command and the treat, and be sure to be really patient, it takes some time and that is absolutely fine. Once you're there, reward your pet every time it earned that treat. You need to get it to trust you!

Last but not least, remember that portion control is key. In many cases, even if treats are homemade, they are still pretty high in calories, and depending on the ingredients you choose, it may also have a relatively large content of fat and carbohydrates. To know how many treats you can give to your little one, you can keep track of an approximate daily intake of all the nutrients it is getting, which you can do by writing down your go-to ingredients, and how much you use of each one of them. Then, take a look at their nutritional and calorie content and add those up. Now you can compare that to your pet's ideal intake and introduce the right amount of treats.

Depending on the type of treat you prepare, you can store them at room temperature, in the fridge or freezer, and even make them right before using them. Like all other meals, the way you prepare and store them is completely up to you, and you should always prioritize your pet's safety when making that call.

Homemade Treats for Dogs and Cats

In this section, I will share some ideas for treats you can prepare for your furry friend. Most of them can be used for almost any dog or cat, regardless of their age and health conditions, and they will certainly love it, so give them a go, I promise they are all really easy, tasty, and nutritious.

Liver Treats

- Ingredients. 1 ½ pounds of beef or chicken liver, 2 eggs, and ½ cup of plain whole grain oat flour.

- Preparation.

    a. Preheat your oven at 350 °F, and while that happens cover a tray with parchment paper.

    b. Cut the liver into smaller pieces and then put them into a blender or food processor until you get really small pieces.

    c. Add the flour and eggs, and then process it again until you get a homogenous mixture.

    d. Spread on the tray and bake for 15 minutes or until fully cooked.

    e. Let it cool down and then cut it into smaller pieces, preferably into a size that suits your pet's mouth.

Carrot Treats

- Ingredients. 1 cup of shredded carrot, 1 cup of unsweetened applesauce, 2 cups of whole grain oat flour, a tablespoon of chopped parsley, and one tablespoon of flax meal –this is optional. If you want to give this recipe a twist, you can substitute the carrot by sweet potato and drop the flax meal.

- Preparation.

    a. Preheat your oven at 350 °F, and while that happens cover a tray with parchment paper.

    b. Take the flax and add 3 tablespoons of water to it. Set aside for a couple of minutes.

    c. Mix the carrots, parsley, applesauce, and oat flour. Then add the rest of the ingredients in that bowl and mix everything together until you get a uniform dough. If you decide on sweet potatoes, make sure that they are cooked until tender before this step. You can do so by boiling them or microwaving them for about 7 minutes.

    d. Transfer all the mixture to your tray and try to sparse it as evenly as possible. Another optional step is to use a cookie cutter to make smaller pieces, but you can just cut them with a knife as well.

    e. Bake for an hour or until fully cooked and crunchy. Now they're ready for your pet to try!

Tuna Treats

- Ingredients. Just get a can of tuna, 1 egg, a cup of oat flour—you can also use whole wheat flour—and a banana.

- Preparation.

    a. Preheat your oven to 350 °F, and cover a tray with parchment paper.

    b. First, mash the banana until you get a soft and uniform paste.

c. Add the rest of the ingredients to the mashed banana and incorporate everything until it looks as homogenous as possible.

d. Spread and flatten the mixture on the tray and bake it for about 15 minutes.

e. Wait for it to cool down and then cut it into small-sized treats. Now they're ready for your pet to enjoy.

Chapter 9:

Pet Meal Prep and Storage

Back in Chapter 3, you learned some tips to help you turn meal prep time into something much easier, entertaining and efficient while preserving the benefits of your pet's dishes. However, there is much more to be said when it comes to this amazing practice, especially because food safety and handling are not to be taken lightly, and even more so when food will be stored for longer periods of time.

Food Safety

Storage and Refrigeration

Most, if not all, of the ingredients you will use to prepare your pet's food requires refrigeration if not consumed right after making it. However, the role that refrigeration plays in your meal prep process will depend on the type of meal you prepare and how long ahead you're planning for.

If your pet is a big meat eater, the safest way to store all sorts of meat is to freeze it until you're ready to cook it. In fact, if you're meal prepping for periods longer than five to seven days, you should definitely store those cooked meals in the freezer to ensure that they don't go bad during that time. In the case of veggies, you can also store them in a sealed container once they're cooked, and you can choose between the fridge and the freezer depending on the amount of time.

When you store your meals in the fridge, you have to make sure that the temperature ranges between 40 °F to 45 °F at most, as this is the optimal temperature for a refrigerator. Meanwhile, frozen foods should be ideally kept at 0 °F.

As for fresh vegetables and fruits, make sure that you clean them and then store them—preferably in containers as well—at 40 °F to 45 °F too. Some, like carrots and celery, could use some water in the container to keep them from dehydrating due to cold temperatures. Foods like cooked rice and other cereals, steamed vegetables, or natural treats also do good at this temperature for up to 10 days. The goal of storing food in cold temperatures is to stop or slow down microorganisms from growing, which is the best way to prevent a stomach infection.

Handling Food

Ground rules to handle your pet's food are not too different from those of our own meals. For instance, you must always wash your hands and always use clean utensils when cooking for your pet. However, there is no harm in going over a few tips I told you about earlier.

Other than doing everything in a way that is as clean as possible, it's really important that you assign utensils that are specific to raw meat, as it is more likely to act as a vector of infectious diseases, especially before cooking. Assigned cutting boards are a must, and you must avoid using those to cut veggies or other foods in order to prevent cross-contamination, which is a process in which microorganisms go from one type of food to another that is completely different. On that same note, avoid rinsing meat under the faucet, because this causes water to splash nearby objects and ingredients, meaning another high risk for cross-contamination.

Storing at Room Temperature

There are certainly a variety of ingredients that you don't need to refrigerate or freeze, but nonetheless require some measures to preserve their freshness and avoid microbial growth. Such is the case of cereals, seeds, oils, and grains, all of which are important components of all pets' diets.

To store these ingredients right, you will need to properly clean your hermetic containers and preferably assign specific containers to each ingredient to reduce the risk of contamination. Once they are clean and completely dry, you can proceed to pour the ingredients in, always making sure that the lid seals completely to prevent environmental damage from making your food go bad. Some extra measures you can take to make these ingredients last for longer are to keep the containers in cool places, away from the sunlight. This will slow down the growth of dangerous microbes in case the ingredient itself contains any. Now that you've learned about recipes, tips, and tricks, you're probably wondering about the evidence that proves that this lifestyle is the way to go, or how they even establish what is good for your pet in the first place. Why don't we talk a little bit about the role of science in our pets' nutrition?

Chapter 10:

The Science of Pet Nutrition

You have made it this far, so by now there's no doubt that you know pet nutrition is to be taken just as seriously as our own. Like I said in the first few chapters of this book, a complete diet should always include all types of macronutrients and micronutrients, meaning an adequate amount of protein, carbohydrates, and fats, along with enough vitamins and minerals. Your pet's digestive system is innately designed to break down said nutrients and fuel their body so that they can stay healthy and active, while always respecting its lifestyle and energy demands.

Because of how complex this topic can be, there are several organizations in charge of studying and regulating pet nutrition. The American College of Veterinary Nutrition and the Association of American Feed Control Officials (AAFCO) are two of the most important institutions that work on this subject, and they have established some criteria that pet food should follow in order to be considered balanced and healthy. To keep things simple, we're going to stick to the part of this information that tells us what we need to keep an eye on when trying to meet adequate pet nourishment.

For instance, both the American College of Veterinary Nutrition and the AAFCO state that factors to consider when creating a proper diet for your pet include growth, age group, level of activity, reproduction, and medical or behavioral conditions. I know you're not a stranger to this information because we've been seeing in the past chapters, but putting an emphasis on how important these factors are is a must.

Along the same lines, note that the AAFCO also stated the six types of nutrients required for pets to thrive. The list consists of protein, fat, carbohydrates, vitamins, minerals, and water. If you recall, earlier in the book I explained what these are in more detail, so feel free to head back to Chapter 1 for more information on that matter. In this chapter, you will learn about how commercial dog food is made and why it is considered to perfectly meet all of your pet's nutritional needs. I will also expand on how exactly you can aim at developing a similar food composition through natural and fresh ingredients, without the use of additives.

Other topics we will go into further detail include the role of additives such as artificial flavors, and other elements that are important in the composition of both regular and specialized diets. Last, but not least, I'm going to wrap up the chapter—and the book—by debunking some popular myths and misconceptions about dog nutrition that you may find very interesting. Let's get to it.

Scientific Foundations of Pet Nutrition

Although the goal of this book is for you to create a fantastic homemade diet, it is important that you understand more about the foundations of regular pet foods so that you know what science has established as "the optimal way to feed your pet," and then make it better. To get off to a good start, here are some concepts you may have already seen or heard about, only this time you'll see what they mean and why they are so important.

Protein Quality

Remember how in Chapter 1 I told you about high-quality protein? Here's what I mean by that. Protein, a primary source of energy for domestic animals like cats and dogs, is degraded into amino acids, which are ultimately used to fuel your pet's body, providing it with energy and helping it renew cells and build muscle. Protein quality is defined as the amount of ingested protein that is degraded into essential amino acids to enter metabolic pathways.

Ideally, you would want to provide a predominantly carnivore pet with large amounts of essential amino acids—meaning those must be forcibly obtained through food as they cannot be made by the body—which comes from lean protein sources for the most part. These are considered high-quality proteins because they are rich in valuable amino acids and have lower calorie content, plus they tend to be easily available and have a good taste. As opposed to these products, low-quality protein is found in foods that aren't an easy source of essential amino acids and, rather than that, are rich in other molecules that make it harder for the body to absorb and break down whatever protein they could provide. Some examples are chicken skin or fatty meat.

Protein in Commercial Pet Food

As I have said earlier, all pets need high-quality protein in their food, although the percentage of it will depend on certain physiological factors of your pet. Commercial pet food is supposed to provide all pets with the ideal amount of all nutrients, which in many cases are protein-based. Regularly, the ideal amount of protein for domestic carnivore animals like dogs and cats is set between 20% and 40%, although you can go a little above that depending on your pet's requirements. Meanwhile, for other small mammals, protein should be at least 16% of their daily intake, with about 5% of fat to better up its absorption. In the case of ferrets, the advised amount is more similar to that of dogs than it is to other smaller animals, set at 35%, particularly during the early stages of life. These specifications are clear proof of how important protein content is for our fur babies, but what exactly does it do?

The Role of Protein in Specific Health Conditions

The benefits of high-quality protein go way beyond helping your pet feel energized. For starters, we can think about two extremes that may occur way more frequently than you might imagine, which are different weight problems. Processed food is likely to contribute to rapid weight gain, particularly in senior pets or those with underlying conditions. It is also possible that your pet develops certain health issues as a consequence of being overweight, like diabetes, metabolic disorders, or high blood pressure. If a pet is struggling due to some extra weight, high-quality protein can help them reverse the problem, as it will keep it satiated for longer and will reduce their intake of fats and refined carbs.

On the other hand, we have underweight pets. If your furry friend has a tough time putting some weight on, consider that it may be because of many possible issues, like old age, malnourishment, recent infections, or chronic illnesses. In these cases, high-quality protein is meant to help your pet build some muscle, not only because amino acids are crucial for this purpose, but because protein is naturally calorie dense, which helps reach a higher weight goal.

There are also certain stages of life when your pet may need a considerably higher amount of protein. As I have said, older pets need more protein because in this stage the body naturally tends to lose muscle more rapidly, which makes it harder for them to reach and stay at a healthy weight.

However, higher protein content is not always the perfect solution. There are certain health conditions that don't necessarily benefit from protein-based diets, mainly because they involve difficulty processing these nutrients. For instance, the two main organs in charge of degrading protein are the kidneys and the liver, which means that pets that live with kidney or liver disease will have a tough time digesting protein. In these cases, it is better to opt for a high-quality protein diet, but one that is not too protein dense as it could contribute to the amplification of said diseases.

Although a diet rich in protein may be beneficial for weight loss, there are also cases when the struggle to lose weight worsens because of how calorie dense these diets are. Food allergies are also a problem for some pet owners. Although these severe allergies are not that common, it is still very important to keep in mind that there is always a small possibility that your pet may develop some sort of allergy. There are also certain autoimmune diseases that respond negatively to high-protein diets. Nonetheless, even these pets need at least up to 20% of the protein in their daily meals, meaning that it is all the more important to be very wary of the sources of protein that you include in your pet's dishes.

Nutritional Balance in Pet Food

As you can see, the remaining portion of your pet's meal will be composed of other nutrients, namely carbs and fats. In the case of cats and dogs, you can safely provide them with up to 50% of carbs, although replacing some of that with good protein sources—as long as they don't live with a specific condition that doesn't respond well to higher amounts of protein—could be beneficial as well. Meanwhile, fats should stay at around five to six percent.

Smaller mammals like rabbits, guinea pigs, and hamsters seem to be much better at instinctively knowing how to manage their carbohydrate intake. For this reason, if you have decided to stick to a "homemade" diet for them, you can just go ahead and provide them with their favorite veggies and fruits, which are the best source of carbs for them. This is also the best source of fiber, so it contributes greatly to better gut help. On the other hand, commercial food often consists of pellets or grains, which tend to be very calorie dense and far less tasty. In many cases, this type of food leads to obesity and gastrointestinal issues, which is yet another reason to opt for homemade natural diets.

A common misconception regarding small mammals is that they can thrive on nothing but leafy greens, but that is a big mistake. See, the thing is that these foods don't provide enough calories, nor do they contain the right balance of nutrients for your pet. Although these little guys mostly eat veggies, there are certain plants that have way more benefits than others. A diet consisting more of good grass, along with some leafy greens that are dense in nutrients like kale, beet greens, carrot tops, radicchio, dandelion greens and flowers, berry leaves, and cabbage is just what they need to get enough vitamins, minerals, and fiber. Of course, you should also include a smaller amount of other foods, like fruits, pea pods, or carrots.

Although the majority of the available information about pet food is centered around protein, there are definitely some facts about the role of other nutrients in specific health conditions that are worth addressing. I'm sure we can all agree that one of the most concerning nutrients in the human diet is sugar, and that is something we have in common with our furry friends. Believe it or not, there are plenty of metabolic conditions a domestic animal can develop, such as diabetes, heart disease, or obesity, all of which are heavily influenced by carbohydrate intake, and more specifically daily sugar consumption.

This is when yet another case of specialized diet need comes in. In the last section, I told you about how a diet that is lower in protein can benefit pets who struggle with kidney and liver disease and, similarly, a diet that is lower in sugar and other refined carbs but rich in fiber can help your pet keep metabolic problems under control. This is why knowing all the macronutrients and the portions of them you're giving to your pet is so important. Making small changes in portions of certain foods in their meals could have an enormous domino effect on their health, allowing them to enjoy a life that is as normal as possible. Sometimes actions as simple as changing a single ingredient for another one that is apparently very similar are incredibly beneficial, but more on that in the next section.

Recent Research and Advances in Pet Nutrition

With an overcrowded market of commercial pet food, research on it had been set aside for many years, decades even. Maybe in a way, this led to most pet owners taking whatever pet food was more convenient for their furry friend, regardless of the differences between brands, stages of life, or prices. However, recently there has been much more research done regarding the ideal composition of pet food, and even the relevance of other diets that are not mostly processed diets in the form of brown pellets.

Thanks to this, we are now able to access much more information about different ways to feed our pets. For instance, homemade pet food is now in the spotlight for all the right reasons, from its scientifically proven health benefits to innovative ways to bond with your beloved pet.

Studies have shown that when you include ¼ of natural ingredients in your pet's meal, there is a pretty high chance that you're helping make their life longer by up to 3 years in animals like cats and dogs. This can be achieved even if you only start by introducing some fruit and vegetables on your cat's or dog's plate.

Preliminary research also suggests that synthetic ingredients in processed pet foods, such as additives, preservatives, or artificial flavors have a relatively high probability of triggering allergic reactions. In some cases, they may even cause allergies in pets without any previous history of these problems. This is likely due to the high risk of ingredients in these foods being perceived by the body as allergens, which often happens when an unknown substance is put into the body. As you probably already know, problems like these often show up as sudden itching, dry coat, or rashes. However, some pets are prone to having a more intense reaction, meaning they may experience swelling, trouble breathing, or gastrointestinal problems. Although fresh ingredients also have a small probability of causing allergies, artificial ingredients seem to be a little more problematic.

In a similar take, we now know that digestion and mobility also seem to be heavily influenced by the action of artificial ingredients in store-bought pet food. In fact, not only do ingredients in the formulation of the food itself affect your pet's body, but even the packaging may have something to do with it. In the case of wet food, which is often sold in bags or cans, we know that compounds present in these packages, such as aluminum or lead may cause severe health problems. Pets don't have to be directly exposed to these packages—i.e., Licking food off of the container—to absorb them. These elements make their way to the food, which means when you offer your pet some canned food on a regular basis, they are being exposed to potentially toxic elements that are prone to negatively affect their physical and mental health.

Now, despite the many benefits of homemade diets, it is important to remember the role of cooking methods and nutritional equivalencies. A couple of chapters ago, I told you about some cooking techniques that are better at preserving nutrient integrity for your pet's meal, so here I'm going to go a little deeper into that. The principle of this finding is that even if you use the exact same ingredients to prepare a meal for your pet, you'll be getting different amounts and proportions of nutrients just by changing small details in the cooking process. For example, it has been found that starchy vegetables like potatoes increase their sodium concentrations by up to 20% just by being baked instead of boiled.

Similarly, swapping sweet potatoes instead of regular white ones may increase the calorie intake by over 50%, meaning that choosing one ingredient or another may actually mean a major difference depending on your goals. For instance, if you want your pet to get a lot more energy or put on some weight, they will probably benefit more from sweet potatoes. Meanwhile, if your pet is struggling with an overweight problem, boiled white potato would definitely be a better source of carbohydrates. Actions as simple as cooking ingredients independently or mixed together also seem to be an important detail to consider. It is probably because of these new results that many owners get a little confused when it comes to pet food misconceptions that have been around forever. Since many myths are only now being studied—and sometimes debunked—it is fairly easy to fall into the trap of believing what we have been told our whole lives, so why not talk about some facts you thought differently about? Hey, we have all been there, let's do this.

Common Myths and Misconceptions About Pet Food

There are many foods that aren't bad for our pets, at least not apparently. Here's the thing, our pets will definitely enjoy almost any food that they find tasty, regardless if it is good for them or not. If you think about it, it is pretty similar to our experience with processed foods and "junk food", which doesn't do much for us but tastes good.

For example, many house rabbit owners give their pets too much sweet starchy fruits, like bananas or corn, or maybe things like cereals or their derivatives—i.e., Cookies, bread, or breakfast cereal—which are not good for them. Just like candy for us, taking just a little bit every now and then is not that bad, but introducing them on a regular basis may cause trouble. Because of this, it is important that you understand that when your pet has a homemade diet, their food should be specific to them, and you should avoid giving into their cravings too often in order to prevent further health problems.

Another common misconception is that domestic animals should have a diet just like that of the animals they descended from—that dogs should eat almost the same way wolves do—because although they are referred to as "carnivores," they lean more toward the omnivore side, meaning that not only can they benefit from certain carbohydrates, but they actually need considerable amounts of them. Another example of what debunking this myth can do for your pet's diet lies in the selected sources of nutrients.

For instance, it is believed that cats and dogs can get protein exclusively from meat when in reality there are plenty of protein sources that you can include in their diet to complement their dishes, provide other micronutrients and allow them to taste a variety of flavors. Some options include chickpeas, spinach, lentils, yeast, and brown rice. Byproducts of meat and animal origin products, like marrow, egg or gelatin are also amazing foods for them, which not only nourish them, but also provide additional benefits for their bones, joints, and coat.

Related to this, there's the whole veggie dilemma. Many people think that vegetables are not too important, but that's completely wrong. When you transition to a homemade diet, it is crucial that you include veggies in your pet's food even if it is considered to be more of a meat eater. For many pets who are picky eaters, you may need to introduce each vegetable little by little in order to get your pet to become used to these new flavors that might not be as appealing to them. Fruits and vegetables are definitely the best way to provide vitamins, minerals, and fiber.

On the contrary, we have the case of smaller mammals. As I said in the previous section, many owners believe that things like lettuce, alfalfa, or hay are the best food they can give to their fur babies, but their fame is not entirely well deserved. These foods are not nutritionally dense and are made up of water for the most part, so even though they are not bad for your pet, they can't do a lot for it either.

And last but not least, maybe the biggest and most common myth of all: it is impossible to find a diet that is as good as a commercial food. While it is true that there is a lot of scientific work behind commercial food that is specific for a certain type of pet, it doesn't mean that this is the absolute best way to feed your furry friend. Like most processed products in the food industry, pet food became so popular because it is very practical for the average pet owner. It can't get easier than taking a particular amount of dry food and pouring it into a bowl for your pet to eat. You don't have to think much about how to combine it, how to prepare it, where to store it, or how much of it you should be giving to your pet because it is all standardized and made as simple as it can get. However, you are perfectly capable of creating a diet that is actually good for your pet because no one knows it better than you do!

Regarding homemade diets, there are also misconceptions to unveil. Arguably the main one is the fact that many people think that a bigger volume of food equals a bigger amount of calories. This is completely false! The calorie content is very specific to each food, so while in some cases big bowls of food are very high in calories, this is not always the case. Depending on the nutritional content, you might find that an apparently small serving is actually very caloric, while a bigger plate contains very few calories. This is similar to when you see a comparison between a chocolate bar and a big salad; you can see that a regular-sized candy bar easily has twice as many calories as a salad. Now this applies both to processed foods and to more natural ones, which is why you need to be very careful when it comes to portion sizes and ingredients.

Once you have grabbed a hold of how calories and nutrients work, you're ready to ditch old myths about portion sizes to start focusing on what actually nourishes your pet, in a more calculated way. This is probably one of the most important steps to take when you create your pet's diet. It is all a matter of setting your mind to it and gathering as much knowledge on the subject as you can, consulting with your trusted veterinarian to track your pet's health, and just taking the leap.

Conclusion

Now that you've reached the end of this book, you know that homemade meals can completely turn your pet's life around for the better. A properly tailored diet for your pet is the best way to help them enjoy a happy and healthy lifestyle, while also giving them the opportunity to taste many more delicious flavors and have some fun making these dishes with you. Remember that you can always create your pet's favorite and most adequate version of these meals by just changing up some ingredients, but do make sure that you're tracking your little one's health and needs with the help of a veterinary expert. With this knowledge on hand, you're ready to celebrate the joy of cooking for your furry friend and engage with it while providing it with the best of foods!

Glossary

- **Acidic:** Marked by or resulting from an abnormally high concentration of acid. Having a pH of less than 7.

- **Alkaline:** Of, relating to, containing, or having the properties of an alkali or alkali metal: basic. Having a pH of more than 7.

- **Allergens:** A substance (such as pollen) that induces allergy.

- **Allergy:** Altered bodily reactivity (such as hypersensitivity) to an antigen in response to first exposure. Exaggerated or pathological immunological reactions (such as sneezing, difficulty breathing, itching, or skin rashes) to substances, situations, or physical states that are without comparable effects on the average individual.

- **Amino Acids:** Any of the various amino acids having the amino group (NH2) in the alpha position are the chief components of proteins and are synthesized by living cells or are obtained as essential components of the diet.

- **Byproducts:** Something produced in a usually industrial or biological process in addition to the principal product.

- **Chronic Disease:** A disease (such as asthma, coronary heart disease, or diabetes) that continues or occurs again and again for a long time: a medical condition of prolonged duration.

- **Degenerative Disease:** A disease (such as arteriosclerosis, diabetes mellitus, or osteoarthritis) characterized by progressive degenerative changes in tissue.

- **GMO:** Abbreviation of Genetically Modified Organism.

- **Macronutrient:** A chemical element or substance (such as potassium or protein) that is essential in relatively large amounts to the growth and health of a living organism.

- **Metabolic Pathway:** The sequence of usually enzyme-catalyzed reactions by which one substance is converted into another.

- **Micronutrient:** A chemical element or substance (such as calcium or vitamin C) that is essential in minute amounts to the growth and health of a living organism.

- **Multifactorial:** Caused by or dependent on the interaction of multiple genes combined with one or more environmental factors.

- **Obesity:** A condition characterized by the excessive accumulation and storage of fat in the body.

- **Organic Food:** Of, relating to, yielding, or involving the use of food produced with the use of feed or fertilizer of plant or animal origin without employment of chemically formulated fertilizers, growth stimulants, antibiotics, or pesticides.

- **Overweight:** Weight over and above what is required or allowed.

- **Rodent:** Any of an order (Rodentia) of relatively small gnawing mammals (such as a mouse, squirrel, or beaver) that have in both jaws a single pair of incisors with a chisel-shaped edge. A small mammal (such as a rabbit or a shrew) other than a true rodent.

Appendix

Homemade meals will open your mind and introduce you to a new world of experiences, skills, and solutions you never thought existed, and it is even better than any of us imagined. As this knowledge is becoming more widely available for everyone, it is great connecting with people that have decided to be a part of this fantastic movement, just like yourself, and they are eager to find each other. Getting in touch with these amazing people is a great way to exchange recipes, learn new tips and tricks about homemade diets, and even make some new friends for you and your fur baby. Plus, think about the cuteness overload you'll have when you see all the photos and experiences this community is filled with. For this reason, I have decided to drop a couple of ideas for you to find people who are on the same journey. Check out these online communities you can start with!

Online Communities You Can Join

Two brains think better than one, and what better way to get fantastic suggestions for your pet's homemade meal than from people who do it every day? Because I understand that taking the leap into a whole new lifestyle for you and your pet can be a little scary at first, I'd recommend that you join a couple of online groups where people who have been on this journey share their best tips, experiences, and recipes. You will also find other pet owners that are new to the homemade pet food world, just like you. Check out the communities I dropped below so you can start getting in touch with these amazing people!

Healthy Homemade Dog Food Recipes

Visit their Facebook page:
www.facebook.com/groups/637244453680167/

Homemade Healthy Dog Food and Treats—Homemade Treatment

Visit their Facebook page:
www.facebook.com/groups/390033337791423

Nature's Best The Health and Vitamin Expert, Homemade Pet Food Recipes

Visit their blog at: www.naturesbest.co.uk/our-blog/homemade-pet-food-recipes/

Spunky Junky Healthier Homemade Pet Food

Visit their blog at: www.spunkyjunky.com/blogs/weekly-recipe-homemade-pet-food

Recommended Reading for Further Exploration

Pet nutrition is an immense topic to cover, and I will be the first one to admit that there is always something new to learn. If you are like me and you like to stay informed and know the latest updates about pet health research, you will enjoy some other readings. Right here I leave you with recommended reading you can go to if you would like to learn more about the amazing world of pets, and remember that you can also head to the references provided in this book for more information on what you've learned so far.

Cummings School of Veterinary Medicine

Visit the website: vetnutrition.tufts.edu/browse-all-pet-nutrition-articles/

Clinical Findings in Healthy Dogs Fed With Diets Characterized by Different Carbohydrates Sources

Visit the website:
www.frontiersin.org/articles/10.3389/fvets.2021.667318/full

VCA Animal Hospitals

Visit their selection of articles on pet nutrition:
vcahospitals.com/know-your-pet/topics/nutrition

Hepper Dog Blog

More recipes for dogs with diabetes and weight problems:
www.hepper.com/diabetic-dog-food-recipes/

References

ABC Buffalo. (2017, October 17). *12 human foods that are safe for your cat to eat*. WKBW. https://www.wkbw.com/news/12-human-foods-that-are-safe-for-your-cat-to-eat

Accetta-Scott, A. (2019, July 10). *Feeding rabbits naturally | reduce pellet feed*. A Farm Girl in the Making. https://afarmgirlinthemaking.com/feeding-meat-rabbits-naturally-comfrey/

Adams, C. (2020a, October 28). *7 homemade cat food recipes for senior cats (With Pictures)*. Excited Cats. https://excitedcats.com/homemade-cat-food-recipes-for-senior-cats/

Adams, C. (2020b, October 29). *5 homemade cat food recipes for cats with kidney disease*. Excited Cats. https://excitedcats.com/kidney-disease-cat-food-recipes/

AKC Staff. (2019, May 29). *Human foods dogs can and can't eat.*American Kennel Club; American Kennel Club. https://www.akc.org/expert-advice/nutrition/human-foods-dogs-can-and-cant-eat/

Alexander, H. (2020, June). *What are macronutrients?* MD Anderson Cancer Center. https://www.mdanderson.org/publications/focused-on-health/what-are-macronutrients-.h15-1593780.html

American Heart Association. (2010). *Dietary fats.*. Www.heart.org; American Heart Association. https://www.heart.org/en/healthy-living/healthy-eating/eat-smart/fats/dietary-fats

Animal Care Clinic. (2021, September 1). *5 easy homemade cat food ideas for diabetic cat*. Veterinarian in Junction City | Animal Care Clinic. https://www.animalcareclinicjc.com/news/2021/8/30/5-easy-homemade-cat-food-ideas-for-diabetic-cat

Ardente, A. (2020, September 16). *Pet food ingredient and label guide*. Www.petmd.com. https://www.petmd.com/dog/nutrition/pet-food-ingredient-and-label-guide

AwesomeA. (n.d.). *Homemade pet rat food*. Instructables. https://www.instructables.com/Homemade-Pet-Rat-Food/

Babushka. (n.d.). *Tabby tuna cakes (For Kitty) Recipe- Food.com*. Www.food.com. https://www.food.com/recipe/tabby-tuna-cakes-for-kitty-143858

Bontempo, V. (2005). *Nutrition and Health of Dogs and Cats: Evolution of Petfood*. *Veterinary Research Communications*, *29*(S2), 45–50. https://doi.org/10.1007/s11259-005-0010-8

Buff, P. R., Carter, R. A., Bauer, J. E., & Kersey, J. H. (2014). *Natural pet food: A review of natural diets and their impact on canine and feline physiology*. *Journal of Animal Science*, *92*(9), 3781–3791. https://doi.org/10.2527/jas.2014-7789

Cara. (2020, January 28). *Homemade Kitten Food Health, Home, & Happiness*. Health, Home, & Happiness. https://healthhomeandhappiness.com/raw-homemade-kitten-and-cat-food-recipe-all-meat.html#Chicken_and_Salmon-Based_Raw_Kitten_and_Cat_Food_Recipe

Cosgrove, N. (2021, August 5). *10 Homemade Cat Food Recipes Every Cat Will Love*. Hepper. https://www.hepper.com/homemade-cat-food/

Craig, J. M. (2021). *Additives in pet food: are they safe? Journal of Small Animal Practice*, *62*(8), 624–635. https://doi.org/10.1111/jsap.13375

Dog Child. (n.d.). *Science Backed Benefits of Home Cooking for your Dog*. Dog Child. https://dogchild.co/blogs/learn/science-backed-benefits-of-home-cooking-for-your-dog

Godfrey, H. (2023, January 29). *Is High Protein Good for Dogs? All About High Protein Dog Food - Raised Right - Human-Grade Pet Food*. Raised Right. https://www.raisedrightpets.com/blog/high-protein-dog-food/

Harvard T.H. Chan School of Public Health. (2017, March 21). *Carbohydrates*. The Nutrition Source; Harvard School of Public Health. https://www.hsph.harvard.edu/nutritionsource/carbohydrates/

Harvard T.H. Chan School of Public Health. (2018). *Types of Fat*. The Nutrition Source. https://www.hsph.harvard.edu/nutritionsource/what-should-you-eat/fats-and-cholesterol/types-of-fat/

Harvard T.H. Chan School of Public Health. (2019, February 15). *Vitamins*. The Nutrition Source. https://www.hsph.harvard.edu/nutritionsource/vitamins/

Hearing Dogs for Deaf People. (n.d.). *Safe foods for dogs*. Www.hearingdogs.org.uk. https://www.hearingdogs.org.uk/training-our-puppies/dog-treat-recipes/dog-safe-food/

Hewson-Hughes, A. K., Colyer, A., Simpson, S. J., & Raubenheimer, D. (2016). *Balancing macronutrient intake in a mammalian carnivore: disentangling the influences of flavour and nutrition. Royal Society Open Science, 3*(6), 160081. https://doi.org/10.1098/rsos.160081

Hickson, E., & Irish, E. (2022, February 7). *Foods that are safe for dogs, according to a vet - betterpet*. Betterpet - Advice from Veterinarians and Actual Pet Experts. https://betterpet.com/safe-foods-for-dogs/

Holland, T., & Balial, N. (2023, July 12). *The 7 Best Cat Supplements of 2023*. The Spruce Pets. https://www.thesprucepets.com/best-cat-supplements-555079

The Humane Society of The United States. (n.d.). *Plants and food that can be poisonous to pets*. The Humane Society of the United States. https://www.humanesociety.org/resources/plants-and-food-can-be-poisonous-pets

Jamieson, A. (2023, February 14). *10 homemade cat treats your kitty will love*. Care.com Resources. https://www.care.com/c/easy-homemade-cat-treats/

Lee, L., & Bey, G. (2023, March 2). *26 Common Foods and Liquids That Are Poisonous to Dogs*. GoodRx. https://www.goodrx.com/pet-health/dog/what-foods-are-poisonous-to-dogs

Leicht, K. (2020, December 14). *23 Best Dog Gadgets To Make Fur-Parent Life Easier!* Www.k9ofmine.com. https://www.k9ofmine.com/best-dog-gadgets/

Mackenzie. (n.d.). *Guinea Pig Food Homemade*. Caring for All Pets. https://www.caringforallpets.com/guinea-pig-food-homemade/

McNeil, S. (2019, November 23). *Homemade Diabetic Dog Treats: Diet Tips, Recipes & FAQ's*. Healthy Homemade Dog Treats. https://healthyhomemadedogtreats.com/a-definitive-guide-to-homemade-diabetic-dog-treats/#11--1-chicken%0Aasparagus-and-broccoli-bake-

Morgan, J. (2018, October 11). *The Beginner's Guide to Home Cooked Food for Your Dog*. This Dogs Life. https://www.thisdogslife.co/the-beginners-guide-to-home-cooked-food-for-your-dog/

Mouton Dowdy, S. (2020, August 24). *15 Toxic Human Foods You Should Never Feed Your Cat*. Daily Paws. https://www.dailypaws.com/cats-kittens/cat-nutrition/what-can-cats-eat/foods-toxic-to-cats

Nelson, A. (2022, August 20). *Find Out More About the Nutrients Your Pet Needs*. WebMD. https://www.webmd.com/pets/dog-cat-nutrition

NHS. (2023, April 14). *Facts about fat*. Nhs.uk. https://www.nhs.uk/live-well/eat-well/food-types/different-fats-nutrition/

Pedersen, K. (2019, July 11). *The Pros And Cons Of Homemade Dog Food*. Happy Natural Dog. https://www.happynaturaldog.com/pros-and-cons-of-homemade-dog-food/

Pet Loves Best. (2019, February 8). *How to Feed a Cat with Sensitive Stomach - Recipes Included!* Pet Loves Best. https://petlovesbest.com/cat-with-sensitive-stomach-recipes/#Homemade_Chicken

Picard, C. (2020, January 8). *Here's How to Meal Prep Like a Pro*. Good Housekeeping. https://www.goodhousekeeping.com/food-recipes/a28377603/how-to-meal-prep/

R, B. (2018, January 22). *Supplies for Feeding Raw Dog Food: 7 Accessories I Can't Live Without*. ThatMutt.com. https://www.thatmutt.com/supplies-for-feeding-raw-dog-food/

Randall, S. (2022, March 31). *Homemade Dog Food for Kidney Disease Recipe Video (Quick, Simple)*. Top Dog Tips. https://topdogtips.com/homemade-dog-food-for-kidney-disease-recipe/

Reisen, J. (2017, May 4). *4 Popular Dog Supplements & What They're Used For*. American Kennel Club; American Kennel Club. https://www.akc.org/expert-advice/nutrition/popular-dog-supplements/

San Bruno Pet Hospital. (n.d.). *Nutrition in Small Mammals*. San Bruno Pet Hospital. https://sanbrunopet.com/pet-care-tips/nutrition-small-mammals/

School, C. N. S. at C., & Team, C. N. (n.d.). *Browse All Pet Nutrition Articles*. Clinical Nutrition Service of the Cummings School of Veterinary Medicine. https://vetnutrition.tufts.edu/browse-all-pet-nutrition-articles/

Streit, L. (2021, November 1). *What Are Macronutrients? All You Need to Know*. Healthline. https://www.healthline.com/nutrition/what-are-macronutrients#functions

TIMG. (2019, November 9). *Homemade Bird Seed - How To Make Nutritious, Low-Cost Feed At Home!* This Is My Garden. https://thisismygarden.com/2019/11/homemade-bird-seed/

Tupler, T. (2011, August 4). *What's in a Balanced Dog Food? | petMD*. Petmd.com. https://www.petmd.com/dog/nutrition/evr_dg_whats_in_a_balanced_dog_food

Turner, B. (2021, November 15). *Herbs & Spices for Dogs | Preventive Vet*. Www.preventivevet.com. https://www.preventivevet.com/dogs/herbs-spices-for-dogs

Unleash Your Hound. (n.d.). *7 Common Pet Food Myths...Busted*. Hownd. https://dogslovehownd.com/blogs/hownd/7-common-pet-food-myths-busted

Veterinary Information Network. (2017). World Small Animal Veterinary Association Congress Proceedings, 2017. *VIN.com, 2017*. https://www.vin.com/apputil/content/defaultadv1.aspx?pId=20539&id=8506273

Whitney. (2023, April 6). *How to Prepare a Healthy Homemade Diet for Your Rat*. PetHelpful. https://pethelpful.com/rodents/Homemade-Rat-Diet